Blossoming into Womanhood

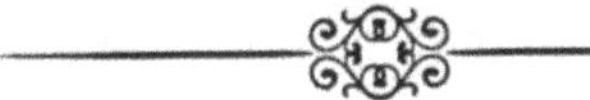

By

Isaac Banahene Amoyaw

TABLE OF CONTENTS

Chapter 1: Understanding Menstruation

What is Menstruation?

Menstruation is a natural process that marks the beginning of a girl's journey into womanhood. It is a monthly cycle that every girl experiences once she reaches puberty. Menstruation, often referred to as a period, is the shedding of the lining of the uterus through the vagina. It may sound daunting at first, but it is an essential part of a woman's life, and understanding it is crucial for maintaining good hygiene and overall well-being.

During menstruation, the body goes through hormonal changes that prepare the uterus for pregnancy. However, if pregnancy does not occur, the body eliminates the lining of the uterus, resulting in bleeding. This process typically lasts for about three to seven days, although it varies from person to person. It is important to note that menstruation is not a sign of sickness but a natural and healthy part of a woman's life.

As a young girl, it is normal to have questions and concerns about menstruation. Educating yourself about this process is essential to ensure you can manage it comfortably. Understanding your menstrual cycle, the signs and symptoms, and the necessary hygiene practices will empower you to confidently embrace this phase of your life.

Maintaining good hygiene during menstruation is crucial for your health and well-being. Changing your sanitary products regularly is important to prevent infections and discomfort. There are various menstrual products available, such as pads, tampons, and menstrual cups. You may need to try different options to find what works best for you.

In addition to hygiene practices, taking care of your mental and emotional well-being during menstruation is equally important. Some girls experience mood swings, cramps, and other physical discomforts during their periods. Engaging in self-care activities, such as exercising, getting enough rest, and eating nutritious foods, can help alleviate these symptoms.

Remember, menstruation is a natural process that should not hold you back from leading a fulfilling life. It is a time to celebrate your womanhood and take pride in the incredible strength and resilience of your body. By understanding menstruation and practicing good hygiene, you can navigate this phase of your life with confidence and grace.

The Menstrual Cycle

Understanding the menstrual cycle is crucial for every girl as it marks the beginning of her journey into womanhood. This chapter aims to shed light on this natural process and provide valuable insights into maintaining good hygiene practices during menstruation.

The menstrual cycle is a monthly occurrence in a woman's body that involves the release of an egg from the ovaries and the shedding of the uterine lining. It lasts around 28 days on average, but this can vary from person to person. During this time, hormonal changes occur, leading to physical and emotional changes that may affect your mood, energy levels, and overall well-being.

It is essential to familiarize yourself with the different phases of the menstrual cycle. The first phase, called the follicular phase, begins on the first day of menstruation. It is characterized by the shedding of the uterine lining, resulting in bleeding that typically lasts for 3 to 7 days. Maintaining good hygiene during this time is crucial by changing your sanitary pad or frequent tampon to prevent odor and infection.

The second phase, the ovulatory phase, occurs around the 14th day of your cycle. This is when an egg is released from the ovaries and is the most fertile time in your cycle. It is essential to be aware of your body's signals during this phase, such as changes in cervical mucus or mild abdominal discomfort.

The third phase, the luteal phase, occurs after ovulation and lasts until the start of the next menstrual cycle. During this time, the body prepares for pregnancy. If fertilization does not occur, the uterine lining sheds, and the cycle begins again.

Maintaining proper hygiene during menstruation is crucial for your overall health and well-being. Changing your sanitary pad or tampon every 4-6 hours, or more often if needed is recommended. Wash your genital area with mild soap and water regularly to keep it clean and prevent any potential infections. Avoid using scented products, as they can cause irritation.

Furthermore, listening to your body and taking care of yourself during your menstrual cycle is essential. Stay hydrated, eat nutritious foods, and get plenty of rest. Engaging in light exercises or practicing relaxation techniques can also help alleviate any discomfort or mood swings.

Remember, every girl experiences her menstrual cycle differently. Understanding your body and maintaining good hygiene practices will help you navigate this natural process with confidence and grace. Embrace your womanhood and take pride in taking care of yourself during this transformative time.

Hormones and Menstruation

Understanding the relationship between hormones and menstruation is essential for every girl entering womanhood. In this subchapter, we will explore the fascinating world of hormones and how they influence the menstrual cycle, as well as provide valuable insights into maintaining proper hygiene during this time.

Every month, a complex interplay of hormones takes place within a girl's body, triggering the menstrual cycle. The two primary hormones involved in this process are estrogenic and progesterone, which are produced by the ovaries. These hormones work together to prepare the uterus for pregnancy. Estrogenic helps build up the lining of the uterus, while progesterone maintains and nourishes it. However, if pregnancy does not occur, the levels of these hormones drop, leading to the shedding of the uterine lining, resulting in menstruation.

While the menstrual cycle can be different for each girl, it generally follows a pattern of around 28 days. During this time, hormones fluctuate, leading to various physical and emotional changes. Common symptoms experienced during menstruation include abdominal cramps, bloating, mood swings, and fatigue. However, it is essential to remember that these symptoms vary from person to person, and not every girl will experience them in the same way.

Maintaining proper hygiene during menstruation is crucial for teen girls and young women. You can ensure a comfortable and healthy period by adopting good hygiene practices. Firstly, changing your sanitary pad or tampon regularly is important to prevent any odor or discomfort. A good rule of thumb is to change your pad every 4-6 hours, or sooner if it becomes saturated. Additionally, washing your genital area with mild, fragrance-free soap and warm water can help maintain cleanliness.

It is also vital to use the right products for menstruation. Choose sanitary pads or tampons that suit your flow and provide adequate protection. There are various options available, such as pads with wings, thin pads, or tampons of different absorbency levels. Experiment with different products to find what works best for you.

Furthermore, adopting healthy habits during menstruation can alleviate discomfort. Regular exercise, a balanced diet, and staying hydrated can help reduce cramps and bloating. Additionally, practicing self-care and managing stress levels can contribute to a more positive menstrual experience.

In conclusion, understanding the role of hormones in menstruation is crucial for girls entering womanhood. Girls can better navigate this natural process by being aware of the hormonal changes that occur during the menstrual cycle. Moreover, maintaining proper hygiene practices during menstruation is essential for teen girls and young women. By following these guidelines, girls can embrace their menstrual journey with confidence, comfort, and good health.

Chapter 2: Preparation for Menstruation

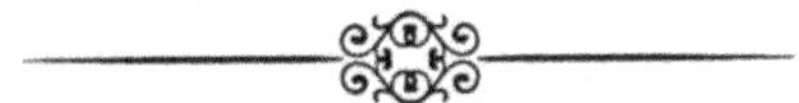

Talking to Parents or Guardians

One of the most important aspects of navigating menstrual hygiene is having open and honest conversations with your parents or guardians. They are there to support you and guide you through this new phase of your life. However, discussing menstruation can sometimes feel uncomfortable or embarrassing. This subchapter aims to provide you with helpful tips on how to approach this topic with your parents or guardians.

First and foremost, remember that your parents or guardians were once young girls too, and they have likely experienced menstruation themselves. They understand what you are going through and can provide valuable insights. Approach the conversation with respect and understanding.

Choose an appropriate time to talk. Find a quiet moment when you and your parents or guardians are relaxed and have time to listen and discuss. You may want to initiate the conversation by saying something like, "Mom/Dad, I have something important to talk to you about. Can we find a time to sit down and chat?"

Educate yourself about menstruation before talking to your parents or guardians. This will help you feel more confident during the conversation and allow you to ask specific questions or seek advice on any concerns you may have. You can refer to the earlier chapters of this book for information.

Express your feelings and concerns openly. Let your parents or guardians know how you feel about starting your period and what worries you may have. They will appreciate your honesty and will be more equipped to offer support and guidance.

Ask questions. Your parents or guardians are your best resource for information about menstrual hygiene. Don't be afraid to ask about different sanitary products, hygiene practices, or any other concerns you may have. They can help you choose the right products and teach you how to use them correctly.

Lastly, remember that your parents or guardians are there to support you. They may have some advice or personal experiences to share that can help ease any anxiety or confusion you may have. Opening this line of communication will strengthen your relationship with them and ensure that you have the necessary support during your journey into womanhood.

In conclusion, talking to your parents or guardians about menstruation is an essential step in navigating menstrual hygiene. Approach the conversation with respect, choose an appropriate time, educate yourself, express your feelings and concerns, ask questions, and remember that your parents or guardians are there to support you. By having open and honest discussions, you can gain valuable insights and guidance that will help you maintain good hygiene practices during menstruation, ensuring a healthy and comfortable experience as you blossom into womanhood.

Gathering Essential Supplies

One of the most important aspects of maintaining good menstrual hygiene is ensuring that you have all the necessary supplies to manage your period comfortably and confidently. In this subchapter, we will discuss the essential items you need to gather before your first period and how to replenish them regularly.

1. Menstrual Products:

Investing in reliable menstrual products is crucial. There are various options available, including pads, tampons, menstrual cups, and period underwear. It's important to experiment and find what works best for you in terms of comfort, absorbency, and convenience. Consider the length and heaviness of your flow when selecting the appropriate product.

2. Extra Underwear:

Having extra pairs of comfortable, absorbent underwear is essential during your period. It's advisable to choose dark-coloured or patterned underwear to avoid visible stains. Keeping spare pairs in your bag or locker can provide peace of mind, especially during long school days or outings.

3. Wet Wipes or Tissues:

Maintaining cleanliness is vital during menstruation. Wet wipes or tissues can help you freshen up, especially when there is no access to water or a bathroom nearby. Look for fragrance-free, biodegradable options to minimize environmental impact.

4. Pain Relief Medication:

Many girls experience cramps and discomfort during their periods. Keep over-the-counter pain relief medication, such as ibuprofen or acetaminophen, in your bag to alleviate any pain. Remember to follow the recommended dosage and consult a healthcare professional if necessary.

5. Disposal Bags:

Proper disposal of used menstrual products is essential for personal hygiene and environmental conservation. Keep small, biodegradable disposal bags or wrappers in your bag to discreetly discard used products. These bags will help maintain cleanliness and prevent any unpleasant odors.

6. Personal Hygiene Products:

Maintaining good personal hygiene is crucial during menstruation. Pack a small toiletry bag with items such as gentle soap, hand sanitizer, and intimate wipes for when you need to freshen up or use public restrooms.

Remember, it's essential to regularly replenish your supplies to ensure you're always prepared. Make a habit of checking your stock of menstrual products and other essentials to avoid any last-minute panic or inconvenience. By gathering these essential supplies and being prepared, you can navigate your period with confidence, comfort, and ease.

Creating a Menstruation Kit

One of the essential aspects of maintaining good menstrual hygiene is having a well-prepared menstruation kit. A menstruation kit is a collection of items that will help you manage your periods comfortably and confidently. In this subchapter, we will explore the essential items you should include in your kit, as well as some additional options that may enhance your overall experience.

The first item you should have in your menstruation kit is menstrual pads or tampons. These are the most common and widely used products for absorbing menstrual blood. It's important to choose the right size and absorbency level that suits your flow. You may want to experiment with different brands to find the one that works best for you. Additionally, consider including panty liners for light flow days or as backup protection.

Maintaining personal hygiene during menstruation is crucial, so make sure to include gentle, fragrance-free wipes or intimate wash in your kit. These will help you stay fresh and clean, especially when you're on-the-go. It's also a good idea to carry a small bottle of hand sanitizer to ensure proper hygiene before and after changing your sanitary products.

To discreetly dispose of used sanitary products, include some sealable plastic bags or odor-lock disposal bags in your kit. These will prevent any unpleasant odors and make it easier to dispose of your used items when a trash bin is not readily available.

Sometimes, unexpected leaks may occur. Consider adding a spare pair of underwear to your kit to avoid embarrassing situations. You can also include some dark-coloured pants or skirts that can easily hide any stains, giving you peace of mind throughout the day.

Lastly, you may want to include some pain relief medication, such as ibuprofen or acetaminophen, to alleviate any discomfort or cramps that may accompany your period. Heat packs or hot water bottles are also great additions to your kit, as they can provide soothing relief when applied to your lower abdomen.

Remember, your menstruation kit is a personal choice, and you can customize it to meet your specific needs and preferences. It's important to have your kit readily available, whether you keep it in your bag, locker, or bathroom. By being prepared and equipped with the right items, you can confidently embrace your menstrual cycle and navigate through it with ease.

Chapter 3: Maintaining Hygiene during Menstruation

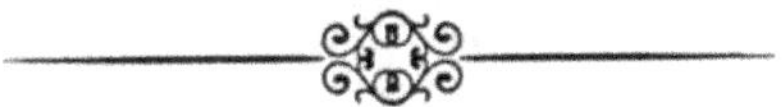

Choosing the Right Menstrual Products

When it comes to managing your period, it is essential to choose the right menstrual products that suit your needs, comfort, and lifestyle. With so many options available in the market, it can be overwhelming to decide which one is the best fit for you. In this subchapter, we will explore different menstrual products and guide you through their pros and cons, helping you make an informed decision.

1. Menstrual Pads: A popular and widely used option, menstrual pads are comfortable, easy to use, and readily available. They come in various sizes and absorbencies, offering protection against leaks. However, some girls might find them bulky or uncomfortable, especially during physical activities like sports.

2. Tampons: Tampons are inserted into the vagina to absorb menstrual flow. They are discreet, allowing you to engage in physical activities without feeling self-conscious. However, using tampons requires some practice and familiarity with your body. It is crucial to change them every 4-8 hours to prevent toxic shock syndrome (TSS), a rare but serious condition.

3. Menstrual Cups: Made of medical-grade silicone or latex, menstrual cups are inserted into the vagina to collect menstrual blood. They are eco-friendly, cost-effective, and can be worn for up to 12 hours at a time. However, using menstrual cups requires practice to ensure a proper fit and prevent leakage. It might take some time to get used to inserting and removing them.

4. Period Panties: This reusable underwear has an absorbent layer built into it, providing both comfort and protection against leaks. They are eco-friendly and easy to use. However, they may not be suitable for heavy flow days or for girls who prefer a more discreet option.

5. Cloth Pads: Like disposable pads, cloth pads are washable and reusable. They are made of soft, absorbent fabric and come in various sizes and patterns. Cloth pads are cost-effective and eco-friendly, but they do require regular washing and drying.

Remember, choosing the right menstrual product is a personal preference. Consider factors such as your flow intensity, comfort, activity level, and environmental impact when making your decision. Finding the perfect fit for you may take some trial and error, but don't be discouraged. Your menstrual journey is unique, and finding the right product will help you feel more confident and comfortable during your period.

Changing Menstrual Products

As girls transition into womanhood, one of the most significant changes they experience is the onset of menstruation. This natural process brings about the need for menstrual hygiene practices that ensure comfort, cleanliness, and overall well-being during this time. One crucial aspect of menstrual hygiene is the choice of menstrual products.

Traditionally, girls have used pads as their primary menstrual product. However, with advancements in technology and a growing focus on sustainability, there are now various options available. Let's explore some of these changing menstrual products and their benefits.

1. Menstrual Cups: Menstrual cups have gained immense popularity among teen girls and young women due to their comfort and eco-friendliness. Made from medical-grade silicone, these cups are inserted into the vagina to collect menstrual blood. They are reusable, reducing waste and saving money in the long run. Menstrual cups can be worn for up to 12 hours, providing long-lasting protection and making them ideal for school or other activities.

2. Period Panties: Another innovative option is period panties. These are underwear specially designed to absorb menstrual blood. Period panties come in various styles and absorbency levels, allowing girls to choose what suits their needs best. They provide a leak-proof barrier, eliminating the need for pads or tampons, and can be reused after washing.

3. Organic Disposable Pads: Organic pads are an excellent choice for those who prefer disposable options. Made from natural materials free from chemicals, fragrances, and chlorine, these pads are gentle on the skin and reduce the risk of allergies or irritation.

4. Menstrual Discs: Menstrual discs are a newer addition to the market. These flexible discs are placed in the vaginal fornix to collect menstrual flow. Unlike tampons, which absorb the blood, menstrual discs collect it, allowing for mess-free removal. They can be worn for up to 12 hours, providing hassle-free protection.

When considering changing menstrual products, it is essential to keep in mind personal comfort, convenience, and individual needs. Finding the perfect fit may take some trial and error, but with patience and exploration, girls can find the menstrual product that suits them best.

Remember, the goal is to feel confident and empowered during menstruation. By embracing these changing menstrual products, girls can easily navigate their menstrual hygiene journey and make choices that align with their values and lifestyle.

Disposal of Menstrual Waste

Proper disposal of menstrual waste is an essential part of maintaining good hygiene during menstruation. It not only ensures our own well-being but also contributes to a cleaner and healthier environment. In this subchapter, we will explore different methods of disposing menstrual waste and highlight the importance of responsible waste management.

One of the most common methods of disposing menstrual waste is using disposable sanitary pads. These pads are designed to absorb menstrual blood and come with an adhesive backing those sticks to your underwear. After use, it is crucial to remove the pad carefully and wrap it in the provided wrapper or a piece of toilet paper. This step ensures that the blood does not encounter other waste and minimizes the risk of spreading infections. Once wrapped, the pad can be disposed of in a trash bin. Remember not to flush sanitary pads down the toilet as they can cause blockages in the sewage system.

For those using tampons, proper disposal is equally important. After removing a used tampon, it is advisable to wrap it in toilet paper or tissue before disposing it in a trash bin. Some tampons come with a biodegradable wrapper that can be used for disposal as well. Never flush tampons down the toilet, as they can cause clogs and damage to the plumbing system.

An eco-friendly alternative to disposable menstrual products is the use of reusable cloth pads or menstrual cups. These products are becoming increasingly popular due to their cost-effectiveness and reduced environmental impact. With reusable cloth pads, proper disposal involves rinsing them with cold water to remove any blood, followed by washing them with soap. Menstrual on the other hand, cups need to be emptied into the toilet or sink and rinsed thoroughly before reinsertion.

Regardless of the method you choose, it is crucial to remember the importance of responsible waste management. Menstrual waste should never be littered or disposed of in public spaces. This not only creates an unhygienic environment but also poses health risks to others. By disposing of menstrual waste responsibly, we contribute to a cleaner and safer world for ourselves and future generations.

In conclusion, the proper disposal of menstrual waste is an integral part of maintaining good hygiene during menstruation. Whether using disposable pads, tampons, or eco-friendly alternatives, wrapping and disposing of them in a trash bin is crucial. Never flush menstrual products down the toilet, as it can lead to plumbing issues. By practicing responsible waste management, we not only take care of our own well-being but also contribute to a cleaner and healthier environment.

Chapter 4: Managing Menstrual Pain and Discomfort

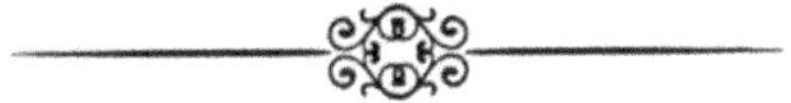

Understanding Menstrual Cramps

Menstrual cramps, also known as dysmenorrhea, are a common and often uncomfortable experience that many girls and young women face during their menstrual cycle. Understanding what causes these cramps and how to manage them effectively is important, as it can greatly impact your overall well-being and daily activities.

During menstruation, the uterus contracts to shed its lining, allowing for the flow of blood. These contractions are triggered by hormone-like substances called prostaglandins. When the levels of prostaglandins are higher, the contractions become more intense, leading to menstrual cramps. Other factors such as stress, poor diet, lack of exercise, and hormonal imbalances can also contribute to the severity of cramps.

The intensity of menstrual cramps can vary from mild discomfort to debilitating pain. Symptoms include a dull or throbbing ache in the lower abdomen, lower back pain, and sometimes even nausea, diarrhoea, or headaches. While it may be tempting to curl up in bed or rely on painkillers, there are several natural remedies and lifestyle changes that can help alleviate the discomfort.

One effective way to manage menstrual cramps is through heat therapy. Applying a heating pad or taking a warm bath can help relax the muscles and reduce the intensity of the contractions. Gentle exercise, such as yoga or walking, can also help by releasing endorphins, the body's natural painkillers, and improving blood circulation.

Maintaining a healthy lifestyle can also play a significant role in managing menstrual cramps. Eating a balanced diet rich in fruits, vegetables, and whole grains can reduce inflammation and provide essential nutrients. It is also important to stay hydrated and limit caffeine and sugary drinks, as they can worsen cramps.

In some cases, over-the-counter pain relief medications like ibuprofen or naproxen sodium can provide temporary relief. However, consulting with a healthcare professional before taking any medication is essential.

Understanding your body's menstrual cycle and tracking your periods can help you anticipate when cramps may occur. By doing so, you can plan, ensuring you have the necessary tools like heating pads, pain relief medication, and comfort measures to manage the discomfort effectively.

Remember, menstrual cramps are a natural part of menstruation; every girl and young woman experiences them differently. It is essential to listen to your body, practice self-care, and seek medical advice if your cramps become severe or affect your daily life.

By understanding menstrual cramps and implementing effective management strategies, you can navigate menstruation with confidence and blossom into womanhood while prioritizing your physical and emotional well-being.

Natural Remedies for Pain Relief

Menstruation is a natural process that occurs in the life of every girl and woman. However, it can sometimes be accompanied by discomfort and pain. While over-the-counter painkillers are commonly used for relief, there are also several natural remedies that can help alleviate menstrual pain. In this subchapter, we will explore some effective natural remedies for pain relief during menstruation.

1. Heat Therapy: Applying heat to the lower abdomen can help relax the muscles and relieve cramps. Use a heating pad, hot water bottle, or take a warm bath to soothe the pain.

2. Herbal Teas: Certain herbal teas, such as ginger, chamomile, and peppermint, have anti-inflammatory properties and can help ease menstrual pain. Sipping on these teas throughout the day can provide relief.

3. Exercise: Engaging in light exercises, such as walking or gentle stretching, can help increase blood flow, reduce cramping, and release endorphins, the body's natural painkillers.

4. Essential Oils: Aromatherapy with essential oils like lavender, clary sage, and marjoram can help ease menstrual pain. Mix a few drops with a carrier oil and massage it onto your lower abdomen.

5. Magnesium-Rich Foods: Consuming foods rich in magnesium, such as dark chocolate, bananas, nuts, and leafy greens, can help relax muscles and alleviate menstrual pain.

6. Relaxation Techniques: Practicing relaxation techniques like deep breathing, meditation, or yoga can help reduce stress and promote relaxation, thus easing menstrual discomfort.

7. Hydration: Staying hydrated is important during menstruation as it helps in reducing bloating and water retention, which can contribute to pain. Increase your water intake and opt for herbal teas or natural fruit juices.

8. Dietary Modifications: Avoiding processed foods, excessive caffeine, and alcohol can help reduce inflammation and alleviate menstrual pain. Incorporate healthy foods like fruits, vegetables, whole grains, and lean proteins into your diet.

Remember, every person's body is unique, so it may take some trial and error to find the natural remedies that work best for you. Additionally, while these natural remedies can provide relief, it's always important to consult with a healthcare professional if your menstrual pain is severe or interfering with your daily life.

By incorporating these natural remedies into your menstrual hygiene routine, you can empower yourself to navigate menstruation with greater comfort and ease. Take the time to explore what works best for you, and remember that self-care during your period is essential for your overall well-being.

Seeking Medical Help

When it comes to our health, it's essential to seek medical help when needed. This is especially true when it comes to matters concerning your menstrual cycle. While menstrual hygiene practices play a crucial role in maintaining good health during menstruation, there may be times when you need to consult a healthcare professional for guidance and support.

One of the primary reasons to seek medical help is to address any concerns or issues you may have regarding your menstrual cycle. Every girl and young woman experience her period differently, and it's essential to understand what is considered normal and what may require medical attention. If you are experiencing severe pain, prolonged or irregular periods, excessive bleeding, or any other unusual symptoms, it's essential to reach out to a healthcare professional.

Another reason to seek medical help is to obtain accurate information and advice regarding menstrual hygiene products. With so many options available today, choosing the right product for your needs can be overwhelming. Consulting a healthcare professional can help you navigate through the various options and find the one that suits you best. They can also provide guidance on proper usage, disposal, and maintenance of menstrual hygiene products.

Additionally, seeking medical help can provide you with valuable information about reproductive health and contraception. It's crucial to stay informed about your reproductive system, the changes it undergoes during menstruation, and the various contraceptive methods available. A healthcare professional can guide you through this information, helping you make informed decisions about your reproductive health.

Remember, seeking medical help is not something to be ashamed of or embarrassed about. Your health and well-being should always be a priority, and healthcare professionals are there to support and assist you. Don't hesitate to reach out if you have any concerns or questions. It's better to address any issues early on rather than letting them escalate into more significant problems.

In conclusion, seeking medical help is an important aspect of maintaining good menstrual hygiene and overall health. Whether it's addressing concerns about your menstrual cycle, obtaining guidance on menstrual hygiene products, or learning more about reproductive health, consulting a healthcare professional is a wise decision. Remember, you are not alone in this journey. Reach out for support and empower yourself with the knowledge to blossom into a healthy and confident woman.

Chapter 5: Maintaining Good Menstrual Health

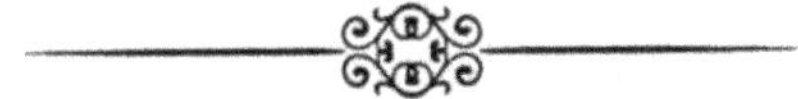

Importance of Regular Exercise

Exercise is an essential aspect of maintaining good overall health and well-being. It becomes even more crucial during menstruation for teen girls and young women. Regular physical activity offers numerous benefits that can positively impact not only your menstrual cycle but also your mental and emotional health.

One significant advantage of engaging in regular exercise during menstruation is the reduction of menstrual cramps. Physical activity promotes the release of endorphins, also known as the "feel-good" hormones, which can help alleviate pain and discomfort associated with menstrual cramps. By incorporating exercise into your routine, you can experience relief from these unpleasant symptoms.

Furthermore, exercise contributes to balancing your hormones, particularly during your menstrual cycle. Hormonal imbalances can lead to mood swings, irritability, and heightened emotions. Engaging in physical activity releases serotonin, a neurotransmitter responsible for regulating mood and promoting feelings of happiness and well-being. Regular exercise can help stabilize your emotions and make you feel more in control during menstruation.

Exercise also plays a crucial role in managing stress and anxiety. Many girls experience heightened emotional stress during their menstrual cycle due to hormonal changes. Physical activity acts as a stress reliever by reducing cortisol levels, the hormone associated with stress. When you exercise, your body produces endorphins, which can help alleviate feelings of anxiety and promote relaxation.

Apart from these menstrual-related benefits, regular exercise has long-term advantages for your overall health. It helps maintain a healthy weight, strengthens bones, and improves cardiovascular health. Physical activity also boosts your immune system, increases energy levels, and improves sleep quality, all of which contribute to your overall well-being.

It is important to remember that exercise during menstruation should be tailored to your comfort level and individual needs. Some activities, such as yoga, swimming, or brisk walking, can be gentle yet effective. Listening to your body and choosing exercises that make you feel good without causing excessive strain is essential.

In conclusion, regular exercise is crucial for maintaining good menstrual hygiene for teen girls and young women. It can help alleviate menstrual cramps, balance hormones, manage stress and anxiety, and improve overall well-being. By incorporating physical activity into your routine, you can experience a healthier and more positive menstrual cycle. Remember to consult with a healthcare professional before starting any new exercise program to ensure it is suitable for you.

Maintaining a Balanced Diet

Eating a balanced diet is essential for overall health and well-being, especially during menstruation. As teenage girls and young women, our bodies go through significant changes, both physically and emotionally. To navigate these changes smoothly and stay healthy, it is crucial to pay attention to our diet and make sure we are getting the right nutrients.

During menstruation, our bodies experience hormonal fluctuations that can lead to mood swings, fatigue, and cravings. While indulging in some comfort foods is normal, it's important to strike a balance and prioritize nutrient-rich meals. Here are some key tips for maintaining a balanced diet during your menstrual cycle.

First and foremost, make sure to include a variety of fruits and vegetables in your daily meals. These colourful foods are packed with vitamins, minerals, and antioxidants that support your immune system and help regulate hormone levels. Opt for leafy greens like spinach, kale, and broccoli, as well as fruits like berries, citrus fruits, and bananas.

Another crucial component of a balanced diet is lean protein. Incorporate lean meats, fish, tofu, beans, and lentils into your meals to provide your body with the necessary amino acids for tissue repair and hormone production. Protein-rich foods also help keep you feeling full for longer, reducing the likelihood of unhealthy snacking.

Whole grains should also make up a significant portion of your diet. Choose whole wheat bread, brown rice, quinoa, and oats over refined grains to ensure you're getting enough fibre, which aids digestion and prevents constipation—a common issue during menstruation.

Don't forget about healthy fats! Avocados, nuts, seeds, and olive oil are excellent sources of monounsaturated and polyunsaturated fats that contribute to brain health and hormone production. These fats also help keep your skin glowing and your hair shiny.

Lastly, stay hydrated! Drinking enough water is vital for maintaining overall health and supporting your body's natural detoxification process. Aim to drink at least eight glasses of water per day, and consider herbal teas or natural fruit-infused water for added flavour.

Remember, maintaining a balanced diet is not about restriction or deprivation. It's about nourishing your body with the right nutrients to support your menstrual health and overall well-being. You can blossom into a healthy and vibrant young woman by making conscious choices and incorporating these tips into your daily routine.

Hydration and Menstruation

During menstruation, it is crucial to prioritize your hydration needs. Staying hydrated not only helps maintain your overall health, but it also plays a significant role in managing your menstrual cycle effectively. In this subchapter, we will explore the importance of hydration during menstruation and provide you with valuable tips to stay hydrated and comfortable during this time of the month.

Why is hydration essential during menstruation? Well, when you menstruate, your body loses fluids through blood flow. This can lead to dehydration if you do not replenish the lost fluids. Dehydration can worsen common menstrual symptoms like fatigue, headaches, and cramps. By staying properly hydrated, you can alleviate these discomforts and promote a healthier menstrual experience.

So, how can you ensure adequate hydration during your period? Here are some tips:

1. Drink plenty of water: Water should be your go-to beverage during menstruation. Aim to drink at least eight glasses of water per day, or more if you engage in physical activities. Sip water throughout the day to maintain a consistent level of hydration.

2. Include hydrating foods: Certain fruits and vegetables have a high-water content and can contribute to your hydration needs. Cucumber, watermelon, oranges, and strawberries are excellent choices to include in your diet during menstruation.

3. Avoid excessive caffeine and sugary drinks: While it may be tempting to reach for caffeinated beverages or sugary sodas during your period, they can dehydrate you. Limit your intake of these drinks and opt for water instead.

4. Herbal teas for hydration and comfort: Sipping on herbal teas like chamomile, ginger, or peppermint can provide hydration while also soothing menstrual cramps. Experiment with different Flavors and find the ones that work best for you.

Remember, every girl's body is unique, and listening to your body's hydration needs is essential. If you experience excessive thirst, dizziness, or dark-coloured urine, these may be signs of dehydration, and you should increase your fluid intake promptly.

By prioritizing hydration during menstruation, you can support your overall well-being and ensure a more comfortable menstrual experience. Stay hydrated, listen to your body, and embrace the power of self-care during your period.

Chapter 6: Dealing with Emotional Changes

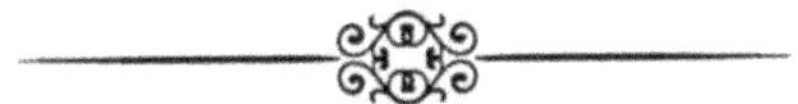

Understanding Hormonal Fluctuations

Hormonal fluctuations are a natural part of being a girl and a woman. These fluctuations occur throughout the menstrual cycle and can have a significant impact on your physical and emotional well-being. In this subchapter, we will delve into the fascinating world of hormones and explore how they affect your body and mind.

The menstrual cycle is governed by a complex interplay of hormones, primarily estrogenic and progesterone. These hormones are produced by your ovaries and play a vital role in regulating your menstrual cycle. Understanding how they fluctuate throughout the month can help you better comprehend your body and manage any discomfort or mood swings that may arise.

The menstrual cycle can be divided into four distinct phases: the follicular phase, ovulation, the luteal phase, and menstruation. Each phase is characterized by different hormonal levels and specific bodily changes. During the follicular phase, estrogenic begins to rise, stimulating the growth of the uterine lining. This phase is followed by ovulation, where an egg is released from the ovaries. Estrogenic levels peak during this time, making you feel more energized and confident.

After ovulation, the luteal phase begins, and progesterone levels rise. Progesterone prepares the uterus for possible pregnancy and can sometimes cause bloating, breast tenderness, and mood swings. If fertilization does not occur, hormone levels drop, leading to menstruation, where the uterine lining sheds.

It is important to remember that hormonal fluctuations can affect everyone differently. Some girls may experience minimal discomfort, while others may have more intense symptoms. It is crucial not to compare yourself to others and to listen to your body. Keeping track of your menstrual cycle using a period tracker app or a simple calendar can help you identify patterns and anticipate hormonal fluctuations. This knowledge can empower you to take care of your body and make informed decisions about your health.

In the next chapter, we will explore various strategies for managing hormonal fluctuations and finding balance during your menstrual cycle. From self-care practices to healthy eating habits, we will provide you with practical tips to navigate these fluctuations and optimize your well-being.

Remember, understanding your body and its hormonal fluctuations is a crucial step in embracing your womanhood. By learning about these changes, you can develop a greater appreciation for your body and its incredible capacity to nurture life.

Coping with Mood Swings

Mood swings are a common and sometimes challenging aspect of our lives as girls and young women. They often coincide with the onset of menstruation and can be confusing and frustrating to deal with. However, it's important to remember that mood swings are a normal part of our hormonal changes and do not define who we are as individuals. In this subchapter, we will discuss some effective strategies to cope with mood swings and maintain emotional well-being during our menstrual cycle.

First and foremost, it's vital to understand that mood swings are not our fault, and we should not blame ourselves for experiencing them. Our changing hormones can impact our emotions, leading to highs and lows that may seem uncontrollable. We can approach our mood swings with greater understanding and compassion by acknowledging and accepting this.

One effective coping mechanism is to practice self-care. Engaging in activities that bring us joy and relaxation can help to alleviate mood swings. Whether it's reading a book, taking a warm bath, going for a walk in nature, or listening to our favourite music, finding time for ourselves is crucial. Additionally, regular exercise and maintaining a healthy diet can have a positive impact on our mood and overall well-being.

Another helpful strategy is to communicate openly with trusted friends, family members, or mentors. Sharing our feelings and experiences with others who understand can provide comfort and support during times of emotional turbulence. It's important to remember that we are not alone in this journey and that seeking help is a sign of strength, not weakness.

Practicing mindfulness and relaxation techniques can also be beneficial in managing mood swings. Taking a few moments each day to engage in deep breathing exercises, meditation, or yoga can help us stay centred and calm. These practices allow us to observe our thoughts and emotions without judgment, enabling us to respond to them in a more balanced way.

Lastly, it's crucial to prioritize sleep and rest during our menstrual cycle. Lack of sleep can exacerbate mood swings, so ensuring we get enough rest is essential. Establishing a consistent sleep routine and creating a peaceful environment can contribute to better emotional well-being.

Remember, coping with mood swings is a journey, and it may take time to find what works best for each of us individually. By implementing these strategies and being patient with us, we can navigate the ups and downs of our emotions with greater ease and grace, ultimately blossoming into confident young women who embrace all aspects of our womanhood.

Seeking Emotional Support

Navigating the ups and downs of adolescence can be challenging, especially when it comes to the changes happening in your body. As you transition into womanhood, it is crucial to recognize the importance of seeking emotional support during this time. Understanding that you are not alone in your experiences and emotions is essential for your overall well-being.

Menstruation can bring about a range of emotions, from excitement to anxiety and even frustration. Feeling overwhelmed or confused as your body goes through these changes is completely normal. This is where emotional support becomes invaluable.

One of the most significant sources of emotional support can be found within your circle of friends. Opening up to your close friends about your menstrual experiences can create a safe space for sharing and understanding. Remember, they may be going through similar experiences, and together, you can support each other on this journey.

Your family members can also serve as a pillar of emotional support. Parents, siblings, or even extended family members can offer guidance, empathy, and advice based on their own experiences. Don't hesitate to reach out and share your thoughts and concerns with them.

If you find it challenging to talk to friends or family about menstruation, consider seeking support from a trusted adult, such as a teacher, school counsellor, or mentor. These individuals are trained to provide guidance and support during your teenage years and can offer valuable advice on hygiene practices and managing emotions.

In addition to seeking support from people in your life, it is important to take care of your emotional well-being through self-care practices. Engaging in activities that make you happy, such as hobbies or spending time in nature, can help alleviate stress and improve your overall mood. Taking time for yourself and practicing self-compassion is crucial during this transformative period.

Remember, seeking emotional support is not a sign of weakness; it is a sign of strength and self-awareness. By reaching out to others and taking care of your emotional well-being, you are empowering yourself to navigate the challenges of menstruation and blossom into a confident, resilient young woman.

In conclusion, seeking emotional support is an essential aspect of navigating menstrual hygiene for teen girls and young women. Whether it be through trusted friends, family members, or other supportive adults, finding someone to confide in can help alleviate the emotional burden of adolescence. Additionally, practicing self-care and engaging in activities that bring you joy can greatly contribute to your emotional well-being. Remember, you are not alone in this journey, and seeking emotional support is a powerful step towards embracing your womanhood and blossoming into the person you are meant to be.

Chapter 7: Managing Menstruation at School

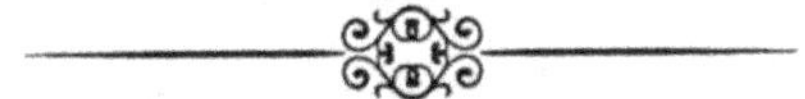

Talking to Teachers and School Staff

In this subchapter, we will discuss the importance of communicating with teachers and school staff about your menstrual hygiene needs. Establishing an open and supportive relationship with them is crucial to ensure a comfortable and stress-free experience during your menstrual cycle.

Firstly, it is essential to remember that menstruation is a natural process that every girl goes through. There is no shame or embarrassment attached to it, and it is vital to approach the topic confidently. By sharing your concerns and needs with your teachers and school staff, you can ensure that they are aware of your situation and can provide the necessary support.

One aspect to consider is informing your teachers about any potential discomfort or pain you may experience during your period. This will allow them to be more understanding if you require additional breaks or adjustments to your class routine. Additionally, if you are participating in physical education or any sports activities, it is crucial to let your teachers know about any limitations you may have during your menstrual cycle.

Another important point to address is the availability of menstrual hygiene products in school facilities. It is necessary to have a conversation with your teachers or school staff about providing access to sanitary napkins or tampons in case of emergencies. By discussing this matter openly, you can ensure that you are prepared for any unexpected situations.

Moreover, speaking with your teachers about your menstrual cycle can also help in planning your academic schedule. Some girls may experience heavy flow or severe cramps during the initial days of their period, which may affect their performance in class. By discussing this with your teachers, you can explore options such as rescheduling exams or adjusting assignments, ensuring that you have a fair opportunity to succeed.

Lastly, if you ever face any discomfort or judgment from teachers or school staff regarding your menstrual cycle, it is crucial to seek support from a trusted adult or counsellor. Remember, it is their responsibility to create a safe and inclusive environment for all students, and any negative experiences should not be tolerated.

In conclusion, talking to teachers and school staff about your menstrual hygiene needs is vital for a positive and stress-free experience during your menstrual cycle. By establishing open lines of communication, you can ensure that your needs are met, and any potential challenges are addressed. Remember, your menstrual cycle is a natural part of being a woman, and you deserve to be supported and respected throughout this journey.

Managing Periods during Classes

One of the most challenging aspects of navigating menstruation as a teenager or young woman is managing periods during classes. The fear of leaks, discomfort, and embarrassment can make this time of the month particularly stressful. However, with the right knowledge and preparation, you can confidently handle your periods while focusing on your studies.

First and foremost, it is essential to be prepared. Always carry a period kit in your bag, containing sanitary pads, tampons, or menstrual cups, whichever option you feel most comfortable with. It is wise to have a variety of absorbencies available to cater to the changing flow throughout your cycle. Additionally, include wet wipes or tissue paper for cleaning purposes and a small Ziplock bag to discreetly dispose of used products.

Timing is crucial when it comes to managing your periods during classes. Try to schedule your bathroom breaks strategically, allowing yourself enough time to change your sanitary product and freshen up. If your school or college has strict restroom policies, speak to a teacher or school nurse about your situation. They are often understanding and can provide the necessary accommodations.

Consider wearing dark-coloured bottoms or invest in period-proof underwear or leak-proof leggings to avoid leaks. These innovative products can provide an extra layer of protection and peace of mind, especially during heavy flow days.

During classes, choose a comfortable sitting position that alleviates any discomfort. If sitting for long periods exacerbates cramps or backaches, consider using a heating pad or taking over-the-counter pain relievers before class. Remember, listening to your body and taking care of yourself during this time is important.

Lastly, don't be afraid to talk to your friends or trusted adults about managing your periods during classes. Sharing experiences and tips can be incredibly helpful in navigating this journey. You may discover new techniques or products that work well for you.

Managing periods during classes can be challenging, but with preparation, timing, and self-care, you can ensure a smooth and stress-free experience. Remember, menstruation is a natural process, and taking care of your hygiene and comfort is paramount. Embrace this phase of womanhood with confidence and pride.

Handling Period-Related Stigma

Menstruation is a natural and beautiful process that signifies a girl's journey into womanhood. However, despite its significance, periods are often surrounded by stigma and misconceptions in our society. This subchapter aims to address the issue of period-related stigma and provide guidance on how to handle it with confidence and grace.

One of the first steps in handling period-related stigma is to educate yourself about menstruation. Understanding the biological process behind it and the reasons why it occurs will help you debunk any myths or misconceptions that may be prevalent in your community. This knowledge will not only empower you but also enable you to educate others who may be misinformed.

It is important to remember that periods are a natural part of life, and there Is absolutely nothing to be ashamed of. Embrace your femininity and be proud of the changes your body is going through. Surround yourself with positive influences and individuals who support and understand menstruation. Seek out friends, family members, or mentors who can provide a safe space for open discussions about periods and related topics.

When faced with period-related stigma, it is essential to respond with confidence and assertiveness. Remember that you have the right to address any disrespectful or insensitive comments or behaviour. Educate others about the importance of menstrual hygiene and the need to break the cycle of stigma. By speaking up and sharing your experiences, you can help normalize conversations around menstruation and empower other girls and women in the process.

In addition, promoting menstrual hygiene practices within your community can also help combat stigma. Organize workshops or awareness campaigns that provide information on proper hygiene practices during menstruation. By sharing knowledge and resources, you can help dispel myths and encourage positive attitudes towards menstruation.

Finally, self-care is crucial in handling period-related stigma. Take care of your physical and emotional well-being during your period. Engage in activities that make you feel good and help alleviate any discomfort. Remember that your period does not define you, and you have the power to embrace your femininity and navigate through this beautiful phase of womanhood with confidence and pride.

In conclusion, handling period-related stigma requires education, confidence, and self-care. By breaking the silence and engaging in open conversations about menstruation, we can challenge societal norms and foster a more inclusive and accepting environment for all girls and women. Let us rise above the stigma and embrace our periods as a symbol of strength and womanhood.

Chapter 8: Menstrual Hygiene and Physical Activities

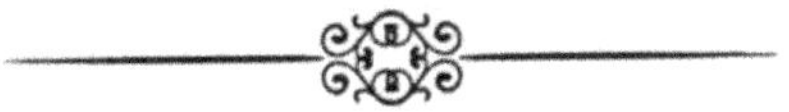

Participating in Sports and Exercise

Staying active and engaging in sports and exercise is not only important for your overall well-being but can also have positive effects on your menstrual health. While it is natural to feel hesitant or concerned about participating in physical activities during your period, it is essential to understand that with the right knowledge and preparation, you can continue to enjoy sports and exercise without any inconvenience.

One of the main concerns girls often have been leakage during physical activities. To prevent this, choosing the right menstrual product that suits your needs is vital. If you prefer pads, opt for those designed specifically for active lifestyles, which offer better protection and absorbency. Alternatively, you may consider tampons or menstrual cups, which are more suitable for sports and exercise, as they are less likely to cause discomfort or leakage.

Maintaining proper hygiene practices during sports and exercise is crucial to avoid any discomfort or potential infections. Before engaging in physical activities, make sure to change your menstrual product and clean yourself thoroughly. If using tampons, remember to change them regularly to prevent the risk of toxic shock syndrome (TSS). Additionally, carry extra menstrual products and wipes with you to maintain cleanliness and freshness throughout your activities.

Another concern girls may have been the impact of physical activities on their menstrual cycle. While intense exercise or sports can occasionally cause irregularities in your cycle, regular physical activity has been shown to have numerous benefits for menstrual health. Exercise helps regulate hormonal balance, reduce menstrual cramps, and improve your mood by releasing endorphins. So, don't be afraid to embrace sports and exercise during your period.

If you feel discomfort or experience severe menstrual symptoms during physical activities, it is essential to listen to your body and take breaks when needed. Stay hydrated, eat nutritious foods, and engage in activities that make you feel comfortable. Remember, your menstrual health should never be a barrier to your active lifestyle, so find a balance that works for you.

In conclusion, participating in sports and exercise is not only possible but also beneficial during menstruation. By selecting the right menstrual products, maintaining proper hygiene practices, and listening to your body, you can continue to enjoy the benefits of physical activity while managing your menstrual health effectively. Don't let your period hold you back from blossoming into the confident, active woman you are meant to be.

Swimming and Menstruation

Swimming can be a fun and enjoyable activity, especially during those hot summer days. But what happens when you have your period? Many girls and young women often wonder if it is safe to swim during menstruation. The good news is that swimming while on your period is perfectly safe and can even provide some relief from menstrual discomfort.

First and foremost, it is important to remember that your period should never hold you back from doing the things you love. However, it is crucial to take some precautions to ensure your comfort and maintain good hygiene during swimming.

Before getting into the water, make sure you are wearing a reliable menstrual product that suits your needs. Whether it's a tampon, menstrual cup, or period-proof swimwear, choose what works best for you. Tampons are a popular choice among swimmers as they are discreet and allow for unrestricted movement.

It's important to change your tampon or empty your menstrual cup before and after swimming to prevent any potential leaks. If you prefer using period-proof swimwear, ensure they are properly fitted to provide maximum protection. Remember to follow the manufacturer's guidelines for usage and care.

Maintaining good hygiene during swimming is essential to prevent any infections. Always rinse off before and after swimming to remove any chlorine or saltwater from your body. Use a gentle, unscented soap to clean your external genital area, and avoid using any scented products, as they can disrupt the natural pH balance and cause irritation.

Additionally, don't forget to bring extra menstrual products with you to the pool or beach just in case you need to change. It's always better to be prepared than caught off guard.

If you feel uncomfortable or experience severe cramps while swimming, it's perfectly okay to take a break. Listen to your body and do what feels right for you. Engaging in light stretches or taking a short walk can help alleviate menstrual discomfort.

Remember, swimming during menstruation is a personal choice. If you feel self-conscious or uncomfortable, it's okay to take a break and resume swimming once your period is over. The most important thing is to prioritize your comfort and well-being.

In conclusion, swimming is a fantastic way to stay active and have fun, even during your period. You can enjoy swimming without any worries by choosing the right menstrual product, practicing good hygiene, and listening to your body's needs. Embrace your body's natural cycle and continue to blossom into womanhood with confidence and grace.

Proper Hygiene Practices for Physical Activities

Staying active and engaging in physical activities is a crucial part of a healthy lifestyle for girls and young women. However, it is important to maintain proper hygiene practices, especially during menstruation. In this subchapter, we will discuss essential tips and guidelines to help you navigate through physical activities while ensuring optimal hygiene during your menstrual cycle.

First and foremost, choosing the right menstrual product for your physical activities is essential. Whether you prefer tampons, menstrual cups, or menstrual pads, select a product that provides maximum comfort and protection. Consider the intensity of your physical activity and choose a product with adequate absorption capacity to prevent leakage.

Before starting any physical activity, make sure to wash your hands thoroughly with soap and water. This simple step helps eliminate any potential bacteria or germs that may cause infections. Additionally, it is crucial to maintain proper body hygiene by taking a shower or bath regularly. Cleanse your intimate areas gently with a mild, pH-balanced soap and avoid using any harsh products that may disrupt the natural balance of your vaginal flora.

During physical activities, it is common to experience increased sweating. Change your menstrual product immediately after your workout or any intense physical activity to prevent odours and discomfort. Carry extra pads or tampons in your bag to ensure you have a fresh one readily available when needed. If you prefer using tampons, remember to change them every 4-6 hours to avoid the risk of Toxic Shock Syndrome (TSS).

Furthermore, wearing comfortable and breathable clothing is crucial during physical activities. Opt for moisture-wicking fabrics that allow proper air circulation and minimize the risk of discomfort or skin irritation. Avoid tight-fitting clothing that may restrict movement or cause chafing. It is also advisable to wear dark-coloured bottoms or patterns that can help conceal any potential leaks.

Lastly, maintaining proper hydration is essential during physical activities, especially while menstruating. Drink plenty of water to stay hydrated and replace the fluids lost through sweating. This not only helps maintain your overall health but also aids in regulating your menstrual flow.

By following these proper hygiene practices, you can confidently engage in physical activities while managing your menstrual cycle. Remember, menstruation should never hold you back from pursuing your passions or staying active. Take care of your body, embrace your womanhood, and continue to blossom into the empowered young woman you are destined to be!

Chapter 9: Menstrual Hygiene and Personal Care

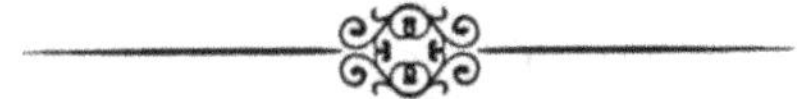

Skin Care during Menstruation

Taking care of your skin is important at any time, but it becomes even more crucial during your menstruation. Your hormone levels fluctuate during this time, which can have an impact on your skin. Understanding how to care for your skin during menstruation can help you maintain a healthy complexion and prevent any potential breakouts or skin issues.

1. Keep your face clean: During menstruation, your skin may produce more oil, leading to an increased risk of acne. Make sure to cleanse your face twice a day with a gentle cleanser to remove dirt, oil, and makeup. Avoid harsh scrubs that can irritate your skin, and opt for products with natural ingredients.

2. Moisturize: Even if you have oily skin, it's important to moisturize to keep your skin hydrated. Look for oil-free, non-comedogenic moisturizers that won't clog your pores. Consider using a moisturizer with ingredients like tea tree oil or salicylic acid, which can help control breakouts.

3. Sun protection: Hormonal changes during menstruation can make your skin more sensitive to the sun. Apply a broad-spectrum sunscreen with an SPF of at least 30 every day, even when it's cloudy. This will protect your skin from harmful UV rays and prevent premature aging.

4. Avoid touching your face: Your hands can carry bacteria and dirt that can lead to breakouts. Avoid touching your face throughout the day, and refrain from popping any pimples or blemishes, as this can lead to scarring and further skin issues.

5. Eat a healthy diet: A well-balanced diet can do wonders for your skin. During menstruation, make sure to include foods rich in antioxidants, such as fruits and vegetables. These can help combat inflammation and keep your skin glowing.

6. Stay hydrated: Drinking plenty of water is essential for maintaining healthy skin. Hydration helps flush out toxins from your body, which can help prevent breakouts and keep your skin looking fresh.

7. Manage stress: Stress can worsen any skin issues you may have during your period. Find healthy ways to manage stress, such as through exercise, meditation, or hobbies that you enjoy. Taking care of your mental health will reflect positively on your skin.

Remember, everyone's skin is unique, and what works for one person may not work for another. Pay attention to how your skin reacts during menstruation and adjust your skincare routine accordingly. By following these simple tips, you can ensure that your skin stays healthy, radiant, and blemish-free throughout your menstrual cycle.

Hair Care and Menstruation

During menstruation, it is essential to focus not only on menstrual hygiene but also on overall self-care, including hair care. Many girls experience changes in their hair during their menstrual cycle, and it is important to understand how to take care of your hair during this time.

Firstly, it is crucial to maintain good hygiene practices during menstruation, as this can have an impact on your scalp and hair health. Regularly wash your hair with a mild shampoo to keep it clean and free from dirt and sweat. However, avoid using harsh shampoos or excessive hair products that may cause dryness or damage to your hair. Opt for a shampoo that is gentle and suitable for your hair type.

During your period, you may notice that your scalp becomes oilier or drier than usual. This is because hormonal changes can affect the production of sebum, the natural oil that moisturizes your scalp and hair. If you experience an oily scalp, consider washing your hair more frequently to maintain cleanliness. On the other hand, if your scalp becomes dry, try using a moisturizing conditioner or hair mask to keep it hydrated.

Another common concern during menstruation is hair fall. Hormonal fluctuations can sometimes lead to increased hair shedding. While this is a normal part of the hair growth cycle, you can minimize excessive hair fall by adopting a healthy lifestyle. Ensure you have a balanced diet, rich in vitamins and minerals, to support hair health. Gentle scalp massages can also improve blood circulation and promote hair growth.

It is important to handle your hair gently during your period. Avoid using heat-styling tools like flat irons or curling wands, as they can cause additional damage to your hair. Instead, embrace natural hairstyles or use heat-free methods like braiding or air-drying your hair. Be mindful of using tight hair ties or accessories that can pull on your hair, causing breakage or discomfort.

Lastly, maintaining good menstrual hygiene is crucial to prevent any infections that may affect your overall health, including your hair. Change your sanitary pads or tampons regularly and ensure proper disposal. Avoid wearing tight-fitting underwear or pants that may restrict airflow to your genital area, as this can create a moist environment that promotes bacterial growth.

Remember, taking care of your hair during menstruation is an important part of your overall hygiene and self-care routine. By adopting these simple practices, you can ensure healthy and beautiful hair all month long.

Maintaining Oral Hygiene

Oral hygiene plays a crucial role in our overall health and well-being, especially during menstruation. As teen girls and young women, it is essential to prioritize oral health to ensure a beautiful and confident smile. This subchapter will guide you through the importance of maintaining oral hygiene and provide valuable tips to keep your teeth and gums healthy throughout your menstrual cycle.

During menstruation, hormonal changes can lead to various oral health issues, such as gum inflammation, bleeding gums, or even canker sores. These issues might occur due to hormonal fluctuations, weakened immune system, or changes in saliva production. Therefore, paying attention to your oral hygiene routine during this time becomes even more crucial.

First and foremost, brushing your teeth twice a day is a fundamental practice that should never be neglected. Use a soft-bristled toothbrush and fluoride toothpaste to gently clean your teeth and gums. Be sure to replace your toothbrush every three to four months or as soon as the bristles become frayed.

In addition to brushing, flossing daily is equally important. Regular flossing helps remove food particles and plaque from between your teeth, preventing the build-up of bacteria that can lead to gum disease and bad breath. Consider using waxed or flavoured floss to make the experience more enjoyable.

During menstruation, it is common to experience dry mouth due to changes in saliva production. Stay hydrated by drinking plenty of water throughout the day to combat this. Drinking water not only helps keep your mouth moist but also aids in flushing out harmful bacteria.

Maintaining a healthy diet is vital for your oral health as well. Opt for nutritious foods such as fruits, vegetables, dairy products, and lean proteins. Limit your intake of sugary snacks and beverages, as they can contribute to tooth decay. If you do indulge in sweets, make sure to brush your teeth afterward or rinse your mouth with water.

Regular dental check-ups are crucial, especially during menstruation. Schedule appointments with your dentist every six months to get professional cleanings and thorough examinations. Your dentist can identify and address any oral health issues before they become major problems.

Remember, maintaining oral hygiene is not only about having a beautiful smile but also about preventing potential health problems. By following these simple yet effective tips, you can blossom into womanhood with a radiant and healthy smile.

Chapter 10: Menstruation and Mental Well-being

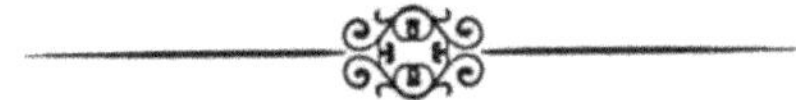

Understanding PMS (Premenstrual Syndrome)

Premenstrual Syndrome (PMS) is a common condition that affects many girls and women during their menstrual cycle. Understanding what PMS is and how it can impact your physical and emotional well-being is important. By recognizing the symptoms and learning how to manage them, you can navigate through your menstrual cycle with confidence and ease.

PMS refers to a combination of physical, emotional, and behavioural symptoms that occur in the days or weeks leading up to your period. While the exact cause of PMS is not fully understood, hormonal changes in your body play a significant role. These hormonal fluctuations can lead to a wide range of symptoms, including bloating, breast tenderness, mood swings, irritability, fatigue, and food cravings.

It is essential to remember that every girl and woman experiences PMS differently. Some may have mild symptoms that are easily manageable, while others may experience more severe symptoms that interfere with their daily lives. By understanding your unique pattern of symptoms, you can take proactive steps to alleviate discomfort and enhance your overall well-being.

There are several strategies you can adopt to manage PMS effectively. First and foremost, maintaining a healthy lifestyle is crucial. Regular exercise, balanced nutrition, and adequate sleep can help regulate hormone levels and reduce symptoms. Engaging in relaxation techniques such as deep breathing exercises, yoga, or meditation can also help alleviate stress and promote emotional balance.

Additionally, keeping track of your menstrual cycle and symptoms can provide valuable insights into your patterns. By using a menstrual diary or a period-tracking app, you can identify when PMS symptoms occur and prepare accordingly. This knowledge will empower you to plan and take care of yourself during those challenging days.

If your PMS symptoms persist and significantly impact your quality of life, it is advisable to seek medical advice. A healthcare professional can provide further guidance and recommend appropriate treatments, such as over-the-counter pain relievers, hormonal birth control, or alternative therapies.

Remember, every girl and woman deserve to feel her best, even during PMS. By understanding and managing your symptoms, you can embrace your menstrual cycle with confidence and continue blossoming into the strong, empowered woman you are becoming.

Self-Care Practices for Mental Health

Introduction:

Navigating the world of menstruation can be a challenging time for teen girls and young women. Alongside the physical changes, it's essential to prioritize mental health during this transformative phase of life. In this subchapter, we will explore self-care practices that can positively impact your mental well-being, helping you blossom into womanhood with confidence and resilience.

1. Embrace Open Communication:

First and foremost, remember that you are not alone in this journey. Reach out to trusted friends, family members, or mentors who can offer support, guidance, and a listening ear. Sharing your experiences and concerns will alleviate stress and promote a sense of belonging.

2. Prioritize Sleep:

Getting enough sleep is vital for maintaining good mental health. During menstruation, hormonal changes can disrupt sleep patterns, leading to fatigue and irritability. Create a soothing bedtime routine, avoid screens before sleep, and aim for at least 7-9 hours of restful sleep each night.

3. Practice Mindfulness and Relaxation Techniques:

Take a few moments each day to practice mindfulness and relaxation techniques. Engage in deep breathing exercises, meditation, or yoga to reduce stress, calm your mind, and enhance self-awareness. These practices promote emotional well-being and help manage any mood swings or anxiety that may arise.

4. Engage in Physical Activity:

Regular physical activity releases endorphins, which are natural mood boosters. Engage in activities you enjoy, such as dancing, cycling, or swimming, to improve your overall mental health. Exercise not only reduces stress and anxiety but also promotes a positive body image.

5. Nourish Your Body:

Eating a balanced diet is crucial for maintaining mental well-being. Consume a variety of fruits, vegetables, whole grains, and lean proteins to provide your body with essential nutrients. Stay hydrated and limit caffeine and sugary foods, as they can impact your mood and energy levels.

6. Engage in Creative Outlets:

Discover and nurture your creative side to express yourself and reduce stress. Engaging in art, writing, music, or any other creative outlet allows you to channel your emotions and thoughts in a positive and productive manner.

7. Set Boundaries and Practice Self-Care:

Learn to say no when necessary and set boundaries to protect your mental health. Prioritize self-care activities that make you feel good, whether it's taking a warm bath, reading a book, or spending time in nature. Remember, taking care of yourself is not selfish; it's essential.

Conclusion:
By incorporating these self-care practices into your life, you'll be better equipped to navigate the challenges of menstruation with grace and confidence. Prioritize your mental health, embrace self-care, and remember that you are a unique individual on a beautiful journey of womanhood.

Seeking Professional Help

When it comes to navigating menstrual hygiene, it is essential for girls and young women to know that seeking professional help is not only acceptable but also encouraged. While most girls may feel hesitant or embarrassed to discuss their menstrual issues with someone, it is important to remember that professionals are there to help and support you through this journey.

One of the first professionals you can seek help from is a gynaecologist or a healthcare provider specializing in women's health. They are trained to address any concerns or questions you may have about your menstrual cycle, menstrual pain, or any other related issues. They can also guide you on different birth control methods, if needed, and help you understand your body better.

Professional help can also be sought from school nurses or counsellors who are knowledgeable about menstrual hygiene. They can provide you with information on how to manage your periods discreetly at school, offer advice on dealing with menstrual cramps, and educate you about the importance of maintaining good hygiene during menstruation.

Additionally, if you experience severe menstrual pain or notice any abnormal changes in your menstrual cycle, it is crucial to reach out to a healthcare professional immediately. They can evaluate your symptoms and determine if there is an underlying medical condition that requires further attention and treatment.

Remember, seeking professional help is not a sign of weakness or something to be ashamed of. It is a proactive step towards taking care of your overall health and well-being. Professionals are there to support you, answer your questions, and provide guidance to ensure you have a positive and healthy menstrual experience.

In conclusion, seeking professional help is an important aspect of navigating menstrual hygiene for teen girls and young women. Don't be afraid to reach out to gynaecologists, healthcare providers, school nurses, or counsellors who can provide you with the necessary information and support. Remember, your well-being is a priority, and seeking professional help is a proactive step towards ensuring a comfortable, healthy, and informed journey through womanhood.

Chapter 11: Menstrual Hygiene and Sustainable Practices

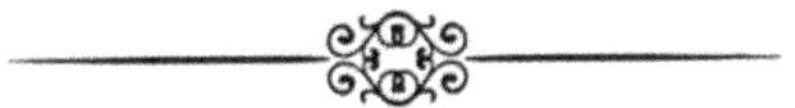

Environmental Impact of Menstrual Products

Menstrual hygiene is an essential aspect of a girl's life, and understanding the environmental impact of the products we use during menstruation is equally important. In this subchapter, we will explore the environmental implications of various menstrual products and how we can make more sustainable choices.

One of the most used menstrual products is disposable pads. While convenient and widely accessible, disposable pads have a significant environmental impact. They are made from plastic and synthetic materials, which take hundreds of years to decompose. Additionally, the production of disposable pads requires a considerable amount of water, energy, and resources, contributing to carbon emissions and environmental degradation. As responsible individuals, we can make a positive change by reducing our reliance on disposable pads.

Another widely used option is tampons, which also have environmental implications. Tampons are typically made from cotton, and conventional cotton production involves the use of pesticides and chemicals that harm both the environment and our health. Furthermore, the plastic applicators and packaging used in tampons contribute to plastic waste accumulation. As an alternative, organic cotton tampons are a more sustainable choice, as they are made from organically grown cotton without the use of harmful chemicals.

An eco-friendly menstrual product gaining popularity is the menstrual cup. Made from medical-grade silicone or latex, menstrual cups are reusable and can last for several years. This significantly reduces waste and the environmental impact associated with disposable products. Additionally, menstrual cups are cost-effective in the long run, and their use promotes a deeper understanding and connection with our bodies.

Reusable cloth pads are another sustainable option. These pads are made from organic cotton or bamboo fabric and can be washed and reused, reducing waste and minimizing the use of resources. They are a comfortable and eco-friendly alternative to disposable pads and tampons.

By choosing sustainable menstrual products, we contribute to the preservation of our planet. Educating ourselves, making informed choices that align with our values and respecting the environment is essential. Additionally, exploring these alternatives empowers us to take control of our menstrual health and well-being.

In conclusion, the environmental impact of menstrual products is a crucial aspect of our hygiene practices. We can minimise waste, conserve resources, and reduce our carbon footprint by opting for reusable options such as menstrual cups or cloth pads, or choosing organic and biodegradable products. Let us take responsibility for the choices we make and blossom into environmentally conscious women who navigate menstruation with care for ourselves and the planet.

Exploring Eco-Friendly Alternatives

In today's world, where environmental concerns are becoming increasingly important, it is crucial for us to explore eco-friendly alternatives in all aspects of our lives, including menstrual hygiene. As young girls and women, it is essential for us to be aware of the impact our menstrual hygiene practices have on the environment and to make conscious choices that promote sustainability. In this subchapter, we will delve into various eco-friendly alternatives that can be incorporated into our menstrual hygiene routine.

The menstrual cup is one of the most popular and sustainable alternatives to traditional disposable pads and tampons. Made from medical-grade silicone or latex, these cups are reusable, comfortable, and long-lasting. By using a menstrual cup, we can significantly reduce the amount of waste generated and the resources consumed. Moreover, with proper care, a menstrual cup can last for several years, making it a cost-effective option as well.

Another eco-friendly alternative to consider is cloth pads. These reusable pads are made from soft, absorbent fabrics such as cotton or bamboo, and can be washed and reused for years. Cloth pads not only reduce waste but also provide a comfortable and breathable option, as they do not contain any chemicals or synthetic materials.

For those who prefer tampons, organic cotton tampons are an eco-friendly choice. Conventional tampons often contain harmful chemicals and toxins, not to mention excessive plastic packaging. Opting for organic cotton tampons not only reduces waste but also eliminates exposure to harmful substances that can have adverse effects on our health.

Additionally, it is important to mention period panties, which are specially designed underwear that can absorb menstrual flow without the need for any additional products. These reusable panties are an excellent option for light to moderate flow days and are available in various absorbency levels.

Exploring eco-friendly alternatives not only benefits the environment but also promotes our overall well-being. By making conscious choices, we can reduce our carbon footprint, minimize waste, and contribute to a healthier planet. So, let's embrace these sustainable options and empower ourselves with knowledge to make informed decisions about our menstrual hygiene practices. Together, we can create a greener and more sustainable future for generations to come.

Spreading Awareness and Advocacy

In today's modern world, it is crucial for girls to be well-informed about menstrual hygiene practices and empowered to advocate for their own well-being. This subchapter aims to equip young girls with the knowledge and confidence necessary to navigate menstruation with grace and dignity. By spreading awareness and engaging in advocacy, we can break the silence surrounding menstruation, dispel myths, and ensure that girls have access to the resources they need to maintain optimal hygiene during this natural process.

Spreading awareness begins with education. It is essential for girls to understand the biological and emotional changes they will experience during menstruation. By providing accurate information about the menstrual cycle, its purpose, and its normal variations, we can empower girls to embrace their bodies, rather than view menstruation as a source of embarrassment or shame. Encouraging open conversations about menstruation at home, in schools, and in the community will help to normalize this natural process.

Advocacy is also a crucial component of promoting menstrual hygiene for teen girls and young women. Girls must be encouraged to speak up about their needs and rights, ensuring they have access to safe and hygienic menstrual products. By advocating for affordable and sustainable options, we can combat period poverty and ensure that no girl is forced to compromise her health and well-being due to financial constraints.

Empowering girls to advocate for menstrual hygiene also involves breaking cultural taboos and stigma associated with menstruation. Girls should be encouraged to challenge harmful beliefs and practices that perpetuate shame and discrimination. By engaging with community leaders, schools, and policymakers, we can create an environment that fosters acceptance and support for girls during their menstrual journey.

Additionally, spreading awareness and advocacy encompass the importance of environmental sustainability. Girls should be educated about eco-friendly menstrual products, such as reusable pads and menstrual cups, which not only reduce waste but also promote long-term cost savings. By choosing sustainable options, girls can take an active role in protecting the environment while maintaining their own hygiene.

In conclusion, spreading awareness and advocacy are vital tools in ensuring proper hygiene practices during menstruation for teen girls and young women. By educating girls, empowering them to speak up for their needs, challenging stigma, and promoting sustainable options, we can create a world where every girl can navigate menstruation with confidence, dignity, and optimal well-being. Together, let's break the silence and embrace the power of knowledge and advocacy to blossom into empowered women.

Chapter 12: Celebrating Womanhood

Embracing Your Body and Changes

As young girls and women, our bodies go through numerous changes, both physical and emotional. One of the most significant changes we experience is menstruation. It's essential to embrace these changes and understand how to care for our bodies during this time. In this subchapter, we will explore the significance of embracing our bodies and provide guidance on maintaining proper hygiene practices during menstruation.

First and foremost, it's crucial to recognize that menstruation is a natural and beautiful process that signifies our transition into womanhood. Instead of feeling embarrassed or ashamed, we should embrace this change and celebrate the amazing capabilities of our bodies. By understanding the menstruation cycle and its purpose, we can develop a positive attitude towards our bodies and the changes they undergo.

Proper hygiene practices during menstruation are vital to ensure our comfort and well-being. Throughout this subchapter, we will discuss various aspects of menstrual hygiene, including the use of sanitary products, maintaining cleanliness, and dealing with discomfort.

Choosing the right sanitary products is crucial to staying comfortable and preventing any potential infections. We will guide you through the different options, such as pads, tampons, and menstrual cups, explaining their benefits and how to use them correctly. Additionally, we will address common concerns such as leakage and odor control, providing practical tips and advice for addressing these issues.

Maintaining cleanliness during menstruation is essential to avoid infections and maintain overall hygiene. We will discuss the importance of regular washing, changing sanitary products frequently, and adopting healthy habits such as washing hands before and after handling sanitary items.

Dealing with discomfort is another aspect that we will address in this subchapter. Many girls experience cramps, mood swings, and other physical and emotional changes during their menstrual cycle. We will provide strategies for managing pain, improving mood, and taking care of our bodies through exercise, stress reduction techniques, and a healthy diet.

In conclusion, embracing our bodies and the changes they undergo during menstruation is essential for our overall well-being. By understanding the significance of menstruation, practicing proper hygiene, and taking care of our bodies, we can navigate this phase of our lives with confidence and grace. Remember, as girls and young women, we are strong and capable of embracing the beauty of womanhood.

Empowering Girls and Women

In this subchapter, we will explore the importance of empowering girls and women, specifically focusing on the topic of menstrual hygiene. Menstruation is a natural and beautiful process that every girl will experience as she blossoms into womanhood. However, it is crucial to have a thorough understanding of hygiene practices during menstruation to ensure our well-being and empowerment.

Firstly, it is essential to recognize that menstruation is not something to be ashamed of or embarrassed about. It is a natural part of being a woman, and it should be celebrated as a symbol of fertility and strength. By understanding this, we can break the societal stigma surrounding menstruation and empower ourselves to embrace this transformative journey.

Education plays a fundamental role in empowering girls and women. By educating ourselves and others about menstruation, we can dispel myths, eliminate taboos, and promote healthy practices. Knowledge about our bodies, menstrual cycles, and hygiene practices equips us with the confidence to make informed decisions about our health and well-being.

Hygiene practices during menstruation are crucial for maintaining good health. It is vital to change sanitary pads or tampons regularly to prevent infections. Proper disposal of used sanitary products is also essential to maintain hygiene and protect the environment. Additionally, maintaining personal hygiene by washing our hands before and after changing sanitary products is crucial.

Empowerment also involves advocating for our rights. We must ensure that every girl has access to affordable and safe sanitary products. Lack of access to these products should never hinder our education, personal growth, or limit our opportunities. By raising our voices and demanding equal access to menstrual hygiene products, we can create a world where no girl is left behind.

Furthermore, empowering girls and women means supporting and uplifting one another. We can create a network of support and understanding by sharing our experiences, challenges, and triumphs. Together, we can break down barriers, challenge societal norms, and empower each other to reach our full potential.

In conclusion, empowering girls and women in the context of menstrual hygiene is about embracing our natural processes, educating ourselves and others, maintaining good hygiene practices, advocating for our rights, and supporting one another. By understanding the importance of empowerment and taking proactive steps, we can navigate the journey of womanhood with confidence, grace, and pride. Remember, as girls, we have the power to change the world and make a positive impact. Let us embrace our femininity, celebrate our uniqueness, and empower ourselves to become the strong, confident women we were meant to be.

Supporting Menstrual Hygiene Initiatives

Menstrual hygiene is an essential aspect of a girl's life, and it is crucial to address the importance of maintaining proper hygiene practices during menstruation. This subchapter aims to shed light on the various initiatives and resources available to support girls in managing their menstrual hygiene effectively.

One of the significant challenges that girls face is the lack of access to menstrual hygiene products. Thankfully, numerous organizations and initiatives are working tirelessly to bridge this gap. These initiatives distribute sanitary pads, tampons, or menstrual cups to girls in need, ensuring they have access to clean and safe options. They also educate girls on the proper usage and disposal of these products, promoting responsible menstrual hygiene practices.

Furthermore, educational programs and workshops play a vital role in supporting menstrual hygiene initiatives. These programs strive to empower girls by providing them with accurate information about menstruation and debunking myths and taboos surrounding it. By educating girls about their bodies and the changes they undergo during menstruation, these initiatives aim to eliminate shame and promote a positive attitude towards menstruation.

In addition to access to products and education, proper sanitation facilities are crucial for maintaining menstrual hygiene. Many initiatives focus on constructing clean and private toilets in schools, ensuring that girls have a safe and hygienic space to manage their periods comfortably. These efforts not only promote menstrual hygiene but also contribute to girls' overall health and well-being.

Furthermore, it is essential to involve the community and create awareness about menstrual hygiene. By engaging parents, teachers, and community leaders, these initiatives aim to break the silence surrounding menstruation and foster a supportive environment for girls. This involves organizing workshops and discussions to address the concerns and questions of both girls and their families, thus creating a space for open dialogue and understanding.

Lastly, it is crucial to recognize and support local entrepreneurs who produce affordable and eco-friendly menstrual hygiene products. These initiatives not only provide employment opportunities but also ensure that girls have access to sustainable and cost-effective options. By supporting these local businesses, we contribute to the growth of the community while addressing the issue of menstrual hygiene.

In conclusion, supporting menstrual hygiene initiatives is of utmost importance for the well-being of girls and young women. By ensuring access to products, education, sanitation facilities, and community support, we can empower girls to navigate menstruation with confidence and dignity. Together, let us strive to create a world where every girl has the resources and support, she needs to blossom into womanhood.

Conclusion: Blossoming into Womanhood

In conclusion, the journey of blossoming into womanhood is a beautiful and transformative experience. As young girls, we face numerous challenges and changes, both physically and emotionally, during this period. However, by understanding and practicing proper menstrual hygiene, we can navigate through these challenges with ease and confidence.

Throughout this book, we have explored various aspects of menstrual hygiene, including the importance of maintaining cleanliness during menstruation, choosing the right sanitary products, and managing menstrual pain and discomfort. By adopting these practices, we can ensure that our menstrual cycles are not hindered by any unnecessary complications.

One of the key takeaways from our discussions is the significance of personal hygiene during menstruation. By maintaining cleanliness, changing sanitary products regularly, and washing our bodies properly, we can prevent infections and promote overall well-being during this time. It is crucial to remember that menstrual hygiene is not just about physical cleanliness; it also encompasses emotional and mental well-being. Taking care of ourselves holistically will enable us to embrace our womanhood confidently.

Another important aspect we explored is the selection of appropriate sanitary products. With the wide range of options available, it is essential to choose products that suit our individual needs and preferences. Whether it is pads, tampons, menstrual cups, or reusable cloth pads, we must understand the pros and cons of each and make an informed decision. By doing so, we can ensure comfort and convenience during our menstrual cycles.

Lastly, we discussed various techniques to manage menstrual pain and discomfort. From practicing yoga and meditation to using heat pads and herbal remedies, there are numerous natural ways to alleviate menstrual cramps and mood swings. By incorporating these techniques into our lives, we can experience a smoother and more enjoyable menstrual journey.

As we conclude this book, I hope that you, dear girls, have found valuable insights and practical advice on navigating menstrual hygiene. It is my wish that you embrace this unique phase of your lives with grace, confidence, and self-love. Remember that menstruation is a natural and beautiful process, and by taking care of yourselves during this time, you are embracing your womanhood and all the strength it brings.

Isaac Banahene Amoyaw

May this book serve as a guide and companion as you continue to grow and thrive, not only during your menstrual cycles but throughout your entire journey of womanhood. Empowered with knowledge and armed with the right practices, you can face any challenge that comes your way. Embrace your femininity, celebrate your uniqueness, and continue to blossom into the incredible woman you are destined to become.